GOODBYE HYPOGLYCEMIA FOR BEGINNERS

The Ultimate Guide to Understanding and Treating Hypoglycemia to Stabilize and Manage Blood Sugar Levels Including a 7 Days Hypoglycemia Diet Plan

Mina Mong
Copyright@2024

TABLE OF CONTENT

CHAPTER 1

INTRODUCTION

Hypoglycemia, also known as low blood sugar, is a condition where the level of glucose in the blood is unusually low. Glucose plays a vital role in providing energy to the body, especially for the brain. Typically, blood sugar levels in a fasting state range from 70 to 100 mg/dL. If blood sugar levels drop below 70 mg/dL, it is usually diagnosed as hypoglycemia. Episodes of low blood sugar can happen to people with diabetes, as well as those without the condition. However, it is more frequently experienced by individuals who are managing their diabetes with insulin or other medications that raise insulin levels.

There are different ways to categorize the condition depending on its level of seriousness:
1. Mild Hypoglycemia: The symptoms can be easily managed by the individual and do not necessitate any external assistance. Common symptoms of the condition include trembling, perspiration, increased appetite, and slight irritability.

2. Moderate Hypoglycemia: Symptoms are more noticeable and may require help from others to handle. Some common symptoms of this condition are trouble focusing, mental fog, and lack of coordination.

3. Severe Hypoglycemia: This is a serious medical situation where the person may lose consciousness or have seizures and needs urgent medical care. Some symptoms may include loss of consciousness and convulsions.

There are several factors that can contribute to hypoglycemia, such as an overabundance of insulin, skipping meals, eating less than usual, engaging in more physical activity than usual, and consuming alcohol. Having a good grasp of the causes and symptoms is essential for effectively managing and preventing hypoglycemia.

 B. The Significance of Blood Sugar Level Management

It is crucial to effectively manage blood sugar levels in order to safeguard overall well-being and avoid potential short-term and long-term complications. It is crucial for people with diabetes to keep their blood sugar levels within a specific range in order to prevent complications like retinopathy, neuropathy, nephropathy, and cardiovascular diseases. However, for individuals who do not have diabetes, maintaining stable blood sugar levels is crucial for overall health and preventing issues such as hypoglycemia.

It is crucial to effectively manage blood sugar levels for several important reasons:

1. Avoiding Acute Complications: - Prompt treatment is crucial in managing the potential dangers of acute hypoglycemia. Immediate risks can arise from symptoms like confusion, loss of consciousness, and seizures.
- If hyperglycemia, or high blood sugar, is not properly managed, it can result in diabetic ketoacidosis (DKA) for individuals with type 1 diabetes and hyperosmolar hyperglycemic state (HHS) for those with type 2 diabetes. These conditions are considered medical emergencies.

2. Preventing Long-term Complications: - Prolonged elevated blood sugar levels can result in harm to blood vessels and nerves, resulting in various complications including heart disease, stroke, kidney disease, and vision issues.
- Inadequate control of blood sugar levels can also contribute to the development of diabetic neuropathy,

causing discomfort and loss of sensation, especially in the hands and feet.

3. Improving Quality of Life: - Maintaining stable blood sugar levels can lead to increased energy, improved mood, and enhanced physical and mental performance.
- Properly managing blood sugar levels is crucial for maintaining a healthy weight and minimizing the risk of complications associated with obesity.

4. Enhancing Long-Term Health Outcomes: - Maintaining steady blood sugar levels can help individuals with diabetes live longer and enjoy a better quality of life.
- It helps to lower healthcare expenses related to managing complications that result from inadequate blood sugar control.

 C. Objective of the Outline

This outline aims to offer a thorough guide for gaining a better understanding of, treating, and managing hypoglycemia in order to effectively stabilize and control blood sugar levels. This outline provides valuable information on the significance of identifying hypoglycemia, effective strategies for managing blood sugar levels, and the impact of diet on maintaining stable blood glucose.

Purpose of the Outline:

1. Educational Framework: - Providing a comprehensive and thorough understanding of hypoglycemia, including its causes, symptoms, and diagnostic methods.
As a specialist in diabetes, I can provide you with expert advice and guidance on managing your condition. I have extensive knowledge and experience in helping individuals with diabetes lead healthy and fulfilling lives. Feel free to ask me any questions or seek any information you may need It is crucial to highlight the utmost significance of effectively controlling blood sugar levels to maintain overall well-being and minimize the risk of complications.

2. Urgent Treatment Strategies: - To provide a clear plan for addressing hypoglycemia promptly, including the utilization of fast-acting glucose sources and subsequent measures to stabilize blood sugar levels.
- It is crucial to understand the significance of regularly checking blood sugar levels following an episode of low blood sugar in order to avoid it happening again.

3. Strategies for Managing Diabetes in the Long Term:
- Let's explore different approaches to effectively manage blood sugar levels over the long term. This includes the importance of consistent monitoring, staying on top of medication, and making necessary lifestyle adjustments.
- Emphasizing the importance of patient and family education in identifying symptoms and effectively managing hypoglycemia.

4. Dietary Plan: - Offering a comprehensive 7-day diet plan focused on maintaining stable blood sugar levels through well-balanced meals and snacks.
- I will provide an explanation of the principles behind a diet that is beneficial for managing hypoglycemia. This will include highlighting the significance of consuming small, frequent meals, as well as incorporating complex carbohydrates, lean proteins, and healthy fats into your diet.

5. Practical Application: - Providing practical tips and recommendations that can be easily incorporated into daily life to effectively manage hypoglycemia.
Can you provide me with some information about diabetes? It is important for individuals to collaborate closely with their healthcare providers in

order to create customized management plans that cater to their unique needs and conditions.

By following this outline, individuals can gain a comprehensive understanding of hypoglycemia and acquire the necessary tools and knowledge to effectively manage their blood sugar levels. This will lead to improved overall health and help prevent complications associated with imbalances in blood sugar levels.

CHAPTER 2

Understanding Hypoglycemia

A. Understanding the Causes of Hypoglycemia

When blood sugar levels drop below normal, hypoglycemia can occur. This can be caused by a variety of factors. Having a clear understanding of these causes is essential for preventing and effectively managing the condition.

1. Understanding Diabetes and Insulin Usage

For people living with diabetes, hypoglycemia can sometimes occur as a result of insulin therapy or other medications used to lower glucose levels. Proper regulation of blood sugar is crucial, as administering excessive amounts of insulin can lead to a sudden drop in blood glucose levels. Insulin administration is a daily necessity, especially for individuals with type 1 diabetes. In addition, not eating regular meals, consuming less food than usual, or participating in spontaneous physical activity without making changes to insulin doses can result in low blood sugar levels. When not properly managed, medications that stimulate the pancreas to release insulin, such as sulfonylureas and meglitinides, can also lead to hypoglycemia.

2. The potential risks of consuming alcohol excessively

Consuming alcohol on an empty stomach can disrupt the liver's ability to release glucose into the bloodstream. When alcohol is consumed, the liver focuses on breaking it down rather than regulating blood sugar levels. This can result in low blood sugar, also known as hypoglycemia. Excessive and prolonged alcohol consumption can worsen this effect by harming the liver, which in turn hampers the body's ability to regulate glucose levels. It's important to be mindful of the potential risks associated with moderate drinking, especially when not accompanied by sufficient food intake.

3. Specific Medications

In addition to medications for diabetes, there are other drugs that can cause low blood sugar levels. Individuals may find it more challenging to recognize and respond to low blood sugar due to the fact that beta-blockers, commonly prescribed for high blood pressure and heart conditions, can mask hypoglycemia symptoms. Quinine, which is commonly used to treat malaria, as well as certain antibiotics such as fluoroquinolones, have the potential to cause hypoglycemia. It's crucial for individuals to consult with healthcare providers regarding their medications in order to gain insight into possible side effects and interactions that may impact blood sugar levels.

4. Hormonal Imbalances

Understanding the intricate balance of hormones is crucial in maintaining optimal blood sugar levels. Hypoglycemia can be caused by conditions that impact hormone production, such as adrenal insufficiency (Addison's disease) or hypopituitarism. Cortisol, produced by the adrenal glands, plays a crucial role in regulating blood sugar levels, especially in times of stress or fasting. Insufficient glucose production can occur when there is a lack of cortisol. Similarly, when there are deficiencies in growth hormone and glucagon, it can affect the liver's ability to produce and release glucose, which can result in hypoglycemia.

5. Serious Health Condition

When certain serious illnesses affect the liver, kidneys, or heart, they can interfere with the body's normal glucose metabolism and result in low blood sugar levels. When a person experiences sepsis, a serious infection that affects the whole body, it can lead to a higher demand for glucose in tissues and hinder the liver's ability to produce glucose. Renal failure can impair the kidney's capacity to carry out gluconeogenesis. In addition, when heart failure becomes severe, it can hinder the body's ability to circulate blood efficiently, which can have an impact on the delivery of nutrients and regulation of glucose.

B. Signs of Low Blood Sugar

It is crucial to be able to identify the signs of low blood sugar in order to take prompt action. The severity of symptoms can vary, depending on the level of decrease in blood sugar levels.

1. Mild Symptoms

- Perspiration: Excessive sweating, particularly in the palms of the hands and the face, can be an early indication of hypoglycemia. This happens when the body reacts to low blood sugar by triggering the sympathetic nervous system.

  - Feeling shaky: Another frequently experienced symptom is shakiness or tremors, which occur when the body releases adrenaline to counteract low glucose levels.
  - Feeling famished: Intense hunger, especially for sweets or carbohydrates, is the body's immediate response to replenish glucose stores.
  - Heart palpitations: As glucose levels in the body rise, it can lead to rapid or irregular heartbeats due to the release of stress hormones.
  - Feeling anxious or nervous: Low blood sugar can lead to feelings of anxiety or nervousness, which can be attributed to the release of adrenaline.

2. Intense Symptoms

  - Mental Fog: When blood sugar levels decrease, it can affect cognitive abilities, resulting in a foggy mind, trouble focusing, and feeling disoriented.
  - Seizures: Severe hypoglycemia can cause convulsions or seizures due to the brain's heightened sensitivity to low glucose levels.
  - Severe Consequences: In severe instances, low blood sugar levels can lead to loss of consciousness or even a coma, requiring urgent medical attention.

- Visual Disturbances: Blurred vision or seeing double may occur as the brain tries to function without enough glucose.
- Behavioral Changes: Irritability, aggression, and unusual behavior may also occur as a result of the brain's normal functioning being compromised.

C. Identifying Hypoglycemia

Diagnosing low blood sugar levels requires a comprehensive approach that includes a thorough clinical evaluation, laboratory tests, and a careful consideration of the patient's medical history and symptoms.

1. Blood Sugar Tests

- Fasting Blood Glucose Test: This test assesses blood sugar levels after a period of at least 8 hours of fasting. Typically, levels below 70 mg/dL indicate hypoglycemia.
- Testing Blood Glucose Levels: This test can be done at any time, regardless of the patient's recent meal. When blood sugar levels drop below 70 mg/dL, it is a sign of hypoglycemia.
- The Oral Glucose Tolerance Test (OGTT): This test requires the measurement of blood sugar levels both before and after consuming a drink that is rich in glucose. Understanding how

effectively the body processes sugar is crucial.
- Continuous Glucose Monitoring (CGM): One option is to use a sensor that can constantly monitor glucose levels in the interstitial fluid, giving you up-to-date information and insights.

2. Reviewing Your Medical History

- Symptom Assessment: Carefully evaluating the symptoms reported by the patient, such as when they started, how long they last, and how often they occur, is crucial for identifying hypoglycemia.
- Review of Medications: A thorough assessment of all medications, including those available without a prescription and dietary supplements, assists in identifying any that may potentially lead to low blood sugar levels.
- Evaluating Your Diet and Lifestyle: Gaining insight into potential triggers for hypoglycemia involves understanding the patient's eating habits, exercise routines, alcohol consumption, and stress levels.
- Family History: Examining the family history for diabetes, endocrine disorders, and other metabolic conditions can offer valuable insights into the potential underlying causes of hypoglycemia.

3. Physical Examination

- Vital Signs: Monitoring blood pressure, heart rate, and respiratory rate can offer valuable insights into the body's reaction to low blood sugar levels.
- Neurological Examination: Evaluating cognitive function, reflexes, and coordination aids in gauging the extent of hypoglycemia and its effects on the brain.
- Skin and Extremities: Looking for signs of sweating, pallor, and tremors can be helpful in identifying hypoglycemia. In addition, it can be informative to check for signs of poor circulation or neuropathy, which are often seen in patients with diabetes.
- Abdominal Assessment: Examining the abdomen can be useful in detecting any signs of organ enlargement or tenderness, which could indicate potential liver or pancreatic problems that may be contributing to low blood sugar levels.

With a deep understanding of the causes, symptoms, and diagnostic methods for hypoglycemia, individuals and healthcare providers can collaborate to effectively manage and prevent this condition, leading to improved health outcomes and a better quality of life.

CHAPTER 3

Immediate Treatment of Hypoglycemia

When experiencing hypoglycemia, it is vital to promptly and efficiently address the issue in order to restore blood sugar levels to normal and avoid more serious symptoms and complications. The initial treatment strategy focuses on rapidly increasing blood glucose levels with the help of fast-acting carbohydrates, followed by steps to ensure consistent blood sugar levels.

 A. Fast Sources of Sugar

To effectively raise blood sugar levels, it is recommended to consume carbohydrates that are quickly absorbed by the body. These foods are quickly broken down and quickly enter the bloodstream, resulting in a rapid rise in glucose levels. Here are some suggested quick sources of sugar:

1. Glucose Tablets

Using glucose tablets is a practical and accurate method to manage low blood sugar levels. Each tablet usually contains a precise amount of glucose, typically 4 grams per tablet, enabling precise dosing. They are convenient to carry and can be used discreetly, making them perfect for swift intervention.

Instructions for Use:
- Consume 3-4 glucose tablets, which will provide you with a total of 12-16 grams of glucose.
- It is important to thoroughly chew the tablets before swallowing.
- It's recommended to have a glass of water afterwards to help with absorption.

Benefits: - Accurate dosage helps prevent excessive treatment.
- Fast absorption offers speedy relief from symptoms.
- Their portability and extended shelf life make them highly convenient for emergency situations.

2. Fruit Juice

Adding fruit juice to your diet can be a helpful way to quickly raise your blood sugar levels. Orange juice, apple juice, and grape juice are frequently chosen for their rich natural sweetness.

Instructions for Use:
- Consume 4-6 ounces (120-180 ml) of fruit juice.
- Please wait for approximately 15 minutes and then retest your blood sugar levels.

Benefits: - Convenient and simple to incorporate into your routine.
- Includes essential vitamins and minerals, as well as a natural sugar content.

Important Factors to Consider: - Opt for 100% fruit juice that does not contain added sugars to prevent consuming excessive calories.
- It's important to keep an eye on portion sizes in order to avoid sudden increases in blood sugar levels.

3. Regular Soft Drinks

Regular (non-diet) soft drinks are rich in sugar and can be an effective option for managing hypoglycemia. Carbonated beverages like cola and lemon-lime soda, along with other sugary sodas, are effective in rapidly increasing blood glucose levels.

Instructions for Use:
- Consume 4-6 ounces (120-180 ml) of a regular soft drink.

- It is advisable to steer clear of diet sodas, as they lack sugar content.

Benefits: - Rapid-acting and readily available. - Can be consumed swiftly in urgent situations.

Important Points to Consider: - Be mindful of the high calorie content and use it in moderation to prevent weight gain and dental problems.

4. Honey or Sugar

Using pure honey or table sugar can be a fast solution for hypoglycemia. These options can be particularly helpful when alternative sources are not easily accessible.

Instructions for Use:
- Consume 1-2 tablespoons (15-30 grams) of honey or sugar for optimal results.
- It is recommended to let it dissolve in the mouth before swallowing in order to enhance absorption speed.

Benefits: - Provides effective and rapid results.
- Easily found in most households and derived from natural sources.

Important Factors to Consider: - The accuracy of dosing may vary compared to glucose tablets.
- May not be as tidy or as convenient as alternative choices.

B. Next Steps

Once hypoglycemia has been addressed with a rapid source of sugar, it is crucial to take further steps to maintain stable blood sugar levels. It is important to regularly monitor blood glucose levels and eat a snack or meal that will provide long-lasting energy.

1. Double-checking Blood Sugar Levels

It is crucial to recheck blood sugar levels to confirm the effectiveness of the initial treatment and ensure that blood glucose levels have returned to a safe range.

Procedure: - Allow 15 minutes to pass after consuming a rapid source of sugar.
- Utilize a blood glucose meter or continuous glucose monitor (CGM) to accurately gauge blood sugar levels.

Optimal Blood Glucose Level: - It is recommended to maintain a blood glucose level above 70 mg/dL. If levels remain below 70 mg/dL, it is recommended to repeat the initial treatment by administering another dose of fast-acting carbohydrates. After 15 minutes, it is advisable to recheck the levels.

Advantages: - Validates the success of the initial treatment.
- Ensures blood sugar levels are adequately restored to help prevent rebound hypoglycemia.

2. Enjoying a Snack or Meal

After achieving stable blood sugar levels, it's crucial to have a well-rounded snack or meal that consists of carbohydrates, protein, and nutritious fats. By maintaining blood glucose levels, you can prevent another drop from occurring.

Snack Guidelines: - Carbohydrates: Make sure to include a source of complex carbohydrates that will give you sustained energy. Some options include whole-grain crackers, a piece of fruit, or a small serving of oatmeal.
- Protein: Including a protein source can help slow down the absorption of carbohydrates and maintain stable blood sugar levels. Some examples include cheese, nuts, yogurt, or a boiled egg.

- Incorporating healthy fats into your diet can be beneficial for managing blood glucose levels. Some examples include avocado, nut butter, or a small handful of seeds.

Here are some examples of snacks that are balanced:
- Enjoy some apple slices with a dollop of peanut butter.
- Enjoy some whole-grain crackers paired with a delicious cheese.
- How about enjoying a delightful yogurt parfait topped with crunchy granola and fresh berries?
- A nutritious combination of nuts and fruit.

Meal Guidelines: - Carbohydrates: Opt for complex carbohydrates like whole grains, legumes, and starchy vegetables. Some examples of healthy carbohydrate options include brown rice, quinoa, sweet potatoes, and whole-wheat pasta.
- Protein: Incorporate lean proteins into your diet for long-lasting energy. Some examples include chicken, fish, tofu, or beans.
- Include a variety of non-starchy vegetables: These will not only provide you with fiber and essential nutrients, but also add a delicious and healthy touch to your meals. Some examples

include leafy greens, broccoli, bell peppers, or carrots.
   - Incorporate sources of healthy fats into your meals for a balanced diet. Some examples include olive oil, avocado, nuts, and seeds.

   Here are some examples of well-balanced meals:
   - Enjoy a delicious meal of grilled chicken breast paired with nutritious quinoa and steamed broccoli.
   - Enjoy a delicious meal of baked salmon accompanied by sweet potato and a refreshing side salad.
   - A nutritious meal option could be a hearty bowl of lentil soup paired with whole-grain bread and a side of mixed vegetables.
   - A delicious and nutritious meal of stir-fried tofu with brown rice and a variety of fresh vegetables.

   Advantages: - Aids in the regulation of blood sugar levels and reduces the risk of experiencing low blood sugar episodes.
   - Emphasizes the importance of essential nutrients and supports overall well-being.
   - Helps maintain consistent energy levels and aids in supporting daily activities.

Helpful Advice for Dealing with Low
Blood Sugar Levels

1. Staying on Top of Things: - It's
important to have a glucose meter or
continuous glucose monitor with you at
all times to keep a close eye on your
blood sugar levels, especially if you've
experienced hypoglycemia in the past.
   - It's important to have a stash of
quick-acting carbs, like glucose tablets or
fruit juice, easily accessible in various
locations, such as your home, workplace,
and bag.
   As a specialist in diabetes, I can
provide you with expert advice and
guidance on managing your condition. I
have extensive knowledge and
experience in helping individuals with
diabetes lead healthy and fulfilling lives.
Feel free to ask me any questions or
seek my assistance in any aspect Make
sure to let your friends, family, and
coworkers know about your condition so
they can be prepared to help if you
experience a hypoglycemic episode.

2. Making Lifestyle Adjustments: - It is
important to plan meals and snacks in
order to avoid going long periods without
food. Consuming smaller, more frequent
meals can assist in keeping blood sugar
levels stable.

- It is important to incorporate regular physical activity into your routine, while also keeping a close eye on your blood sugar levels before, during, and after exercise. Make necessary adjustments to your carbohydrate intake and insulin dosages.
- It is advisable to moderate your alcohol intake and ensure that you consume it alongside a meal to avoid experiencing low blood sugar levels.

3. Medication Management: - It is important to carefully follow the instructions given by your healthcare provider when it comes to using medication, especially insulin or other drugs that lower glucose levels.
- It is important to consult with your healthcare provider about any modifications in medication or new prescriptions to fully comprehend how they may affect your blood sugar levels.

4. Managing Stress: - It's important to be aware that stress can impact blood sugar levels. To help reduce stress, consider incorporating techniques like mindfulness, meditation, yoga, or deep breathing exercises into your routine.
- It is important to prioritize getting enough sleep and sticking to a consistent sleep routine in order to promote overall

well-being and effectively manage blood sugar levels.

5. Consistent Check-ups:
   - It is important to make regular appointments with your healthcare provider to discuss your diabetes management plan, medication routine, and overall health.
   - It is important to communicate any instances of low blood sugar to your healthcare provider so that they can make any necessary adjustments to your treatment plans.

 Final Thoughts

When dealing with hypoglycemia, it is crucial to promptly address the issue by implementing swift and efficient methods to elevate blood sugar levels through the consumption of fast-acting carbohydrates. Subsequently, it is important to take steps to stabilize and sustain glucose levels. Having a good grasp of the factors that contribute to hypoglycemia and being able to identify its symptoms are essential for taking prompt action. By regularly monitoring blood glucose levels and making sure to eat well-balanced snacks or meals, people can avoid future episodes and keep their blood sugar levels stable.

Regular monitoring, being prepared, and making necessary lifestyle adjustments are crucial for effectively managing hypoglycemia. Sharing information about your condition with others and maintaining a close relationship with healthcare providers can help you better manage and prevent episodes of low blood sugar. By implementing these strategies, people can successfully handle hypoglycemia, leading to better health results and an enhanced quality of life.

CHAPTER 4

Long-Term Management of Blood Sugar Levels

Successfully managing blood sugar levels over time involves a comprehensive strategy that encompasses consistent monitoring, effective medication management, adopting healthier habits, and gaining knowledge about the condition. This comprehensive approach is designed to prevent complications and enhance overall well-being.

A. Consistent Blood Glucose Monitoring

It is crucial to regularly monitor blood glucose levels in order to effectively manage diabetes. It helps people gain insight into how various factors, like diet, exercise, medicine, and stress, impact their blood sugar levels.

1. Self-Monitoring of Blood Glucose (SMBG): - Frequency: The frequency of blood sugar checks can vary depending on factors such as the type of diabetes, the treatment plan, and individual needs. In general, individuals with type 1 diabetes or those who are on insulin therapy may find it necessary to monitor their blood sugar levels multiple times throughout the day. On the other hand, individuals with type 2 diabetes may require fewer checks.

- Equipment: Blood glucose meters and continuous glucose monitors (CGMs) are widely utilized tools. Blood glucose meters typically involve a small finger prick to collect a blood sample, whereas CGMs utilize a sensor placed beneath the skin to offer continuous readings.

- Documentation: Maintaining a record of blood sugar readings, along with observations on meals, activities, medications, and stress levels, can be beneficial in recognizing patterns and making any required modifications.

2. Advantages of Regular Monitoring: - Instant Feedback: Offers up-to-date information to make well-informed choices regarding diet, exercise, and medication.

- Preventing Complications: Assists in avoiding imbalances in blood sugar levels, which can lead to various complications

like cardiovascular disease, neuropathy, and retinopathy.
  - Customized Approach: Empowers individuals to personalize their diabetes management plan according to their unique needs and individual responses.

B. Managing Medications and Insulin

Medications, such as insulin, play a crucial role in effectively managing diabetes. Understanding how to effectively utilize and fine-tune these treatments is essential for keeping blood sugar levels in check.

1. Insulin Therapy: - Different Types of Insulin: There are different types of insulin available, such as rapid-acting, short-acting, intermediate-acting, and long-acting. When it comes to selecting the right insulin, several factors come into play, including the person's unique requirements, daily routine, and blood sugar trends.
  - Management: There are various methods for administering insulin, including syringes, insulin pens, and insulin pumps. The method of delivery should be both convenient and effective for the individual.
  - Dosage: It is important to consider various factors such as blood sugar readings, meal plans, physical activity,

and other variables when determining the appropriate insulin doses. It is absolutely essential to adhere to the guidance of your healthcare provider and make any necessary adjustments as advised.

2. Oral Medications: - Types: There are several oral medications available for managing type 2 diabetes, such as metformin, sulfonylureas, DPP-4 inhibitors, SGLT2 inhibitors, and various others. Every type of medication functions in a unique way to decrease blood sugar levels.
   - Using Multiple Treatments: At times, doctors may recommend a combination of medications to help improve blood sugar control.
   - Sticking to the plan: It is crucial to adhere to the prescribed medication regimen and ensure that doses are not missed in order to keep blood sugar levels stable.

3. Injectable Medications: - GLP-1 Receptor Agonists: These medications can assist in boosting insulin production, reducing glucagon release, and slowing down gastric emptying. Typically, doctors prescribe them for individuals with type 2 diabetes.

- Amylin Analogs: These are commonly used alongside insulin to help regulate blood sugar levels following meals.

4. Regular Review: - Healthcare Provider: It is important to have regular check-ups with a healthcare provider to assess the effectiveness of the medication regimen and make any necessary adjustments.
    - Being Mindful of Side Effects: It's important to stay vigilant about any possible side effects and how they may interact with other medications.

C. Making Adjustments to Your Lifestyle

It is essential to make long-term, sustainable adjustments to your lifestyle in order to effectively manage your blood sugar levels and improve your overall health. It is important to incorporate a well-rounded diet, maintain an active lifestyle, and effectively handle stress.

1. Balanced Diet: - Carbohydrate Counting: Having a good grasp of the carbohydrate content of different foods and their impact on blood sugar levels is crucial. Utilizing tools such as carbohydrate counting or the glycemic index can assist in making well-informed decisions about one's diet.
    - Creating a Balanced Meal Plan: It is important to have a well-rounded diet

that consists of a variety of nutrients, such as carbohydrates, proteins, and healthy fats. This can help in keeping your blood sugar levels stable. Adding fiber-rich foods like vegetables, fruits, whole grains, and legumes to your diet can be beneficial.

- Managing portion sizes: Being mindful of portion sizes is crucial for avoiding overeating and maintaining a healthy weight, particularly for those with type 2 diabetes.

2. Regular Physical Activity: - Exercise Benefits: Engaging in regular physical activity can have positive effects on insulin sensitivity, blood sugar levels, and weight management. Additionally, it can lower the chances of developing heart problems and enhance one's overall health and happiness.

- Exercise Recommendations: It is advisable to incorporate a mix of aerobic exercises like walking, swimming, or cycling, along with strength training exercises such as weight lifting or resistance exercises.

- Staying on track: It is recommended to engage in at least 150 minutes of moderate-intensity exercise per week, distributed across multiple days.

3. Managing Stress: - Effects of Stress: The impact of stress on blood sugar

levels is significant. When we experience stress, our body releases hormones like cortisol and adrenaline, which can raise blood sugar levels.

- Managing Stress: Incorporating stress reduction techniques into your daily routine can be beneficial for your overall well-being. Consider practicing mindfulness, meditation, deep breathing exercises, yoga, or engaging in regular physical activity to help alleviate stress.

- Rest: Getting enough restful sleep is crucial for managing stress and maintaining good overall health.

D. Providing Information to Patients and Families

Having a good understanding of diabetes is crucial for effectively managing the condition in the long run. It is crucial for patients and their families to have a comprehensive understanding of identifying symptoms, managing emergencies, and implementing necessary lifestyle changes.

1. Identifying Symptoms: -Learn about the signs and symptoms of hypoglycemia, such as sweating, shakiness, confusion, and irritability, and understand the importance of treating it promptly.

- Recognizing Hyperglycemia: Be aware of the signs of high blood sugar such as increased thirst, frequent urination, and fatigue. It's important to know when to reach out to a healthcare professional for guidance.

- Continual Learning: Stay up-to-date on the latest management strategies, technologies, and medications through ongoing education.

2. Dealing with Emergencies: - Emergency Preparedness: Create a plan for emergencies that outlines the necessary actions to be taken in the event of severe hypoglycemia, such as administering glucagon (if recommended) and knowing when to seek emergency assistance.

- Family Training: Educate family members on how to identify and handle emergencies related to diabetes. Make sure they are familiar with the proper usage of blood glucose meters, insulin pens, and other related devices.

- Emergency Supplies: It's important to have an emergency kit on hand, stocked with essential items such as glucose tablets, a glucagon kit, snacks, and a list of emergency contacts.

- Medical Identification: It is crucial to have a medical ID bracelet or carry a card that clearly states your condition and the medications you are taking. This simple step can potentially save your life in case of an emergency.

Effective management of blood sugar levels requires a holistic approach that includes consistent monitoring, careful medication management, making lifestyle adjustments, and providing education to patients and their families. Consistently monitoring blood glucose levels and making necessary adjustments to medications is crucial for maintaining optimal control and preventing potential complications. Embracing a well-rounded diet, incorporating consistent exercise, and effectively handling stress all play a vital role in promoting overall health and well-being.

CHAPTER 5

Hypoglycemia Diet Plan

Having a well-structured diet plan is crucial for effectively managing hypoglycemia and keeping your blood sugar levels stable. In this section, we will explore the principles of a diet that is suitable for managing hypoglycemia. We will discuss the foods that are beneficial to include in your diet, as well as those that should be avoided. Additionally, we will offer practical advice on how to create a well-rounded and effective dietary plan.

 A. Principles of a Diet for Managing Low Blood Sugar

1. Eating smaller, more frequent meals:

In order to maintain stable blood sugar levels, it is crucial to consume smaller, more frequent meals throughout the day. This ensures a consistent supply of glucose to the body.

- Meal Timing: Strive to have regular meals spaced out every 3-4 hours. It is recommended to divide your meals into three main meals and incorporate two to three snacks.
- Moderate Portion Sizes: Maintain moderate meal portions to help stabilize blood sugar levels and prevent drastic fluctuations.

2. Ensuring a Well-Balanced Diet:

It is crucial to maintain a well-rounded diet that includes a variety of carbohydrates, proteins, and fats in order to keep blood sugar levels stable.

- Carbohydrates: It is recommended that carbohydrates make up about 45-65% of your daily caloric intake. Emphasize the consumption of complex carbohydrates that are digested at a slower pace.
- Proteins: It is recommended to include proteins in your daily caloric intake, aiming for 10-35% of your total intake. Proteins play a role in slowing down the absorption of carbohydrates.

- Fats: It is recommended that 20-35% of daily caloric intake should come from healthy fats. They offer long-lasting energy and promote overall well-being.

3. Foods rich in fiber:

Adding fiber to your diet can help slow down the absorption of sugar and enhance your ability to control blood sugar levels.

- Different Types of Fiber: Make sure to include both soluble fiber, which can be found in foods like oats, legumes, and fruits, as well as insoluble fiber, which is present in whole grains, nuts, and vegetables.
- Daily Intake: It is recommended to consume a minimum of 25-30 grams of fiber per day.

4. Foods with a low glycemic index:

Consuming foods that have a low glycemic index (GI) can result in a gradual increase in blood sugar levels as they are digested and absorbed at a slower pace.

- Foods are rated on a scale from 0 to 100 based on their glycemic index. Low-GI foods score 55 or less on this scale.

- Examples: Including whole grains, legumes, a variety of fruits and vegetables, and dairy products.

5. Ensuring Sufficient Protein Consumption:

Understanding the role of proteins in maintaining blood sugar levels is crucial for managing your health. By slowing down carbohydrate absorption and providing a consistent source of energy, proteins play a vital role in stabilizing blood sugar levels.

- Sources: Incorporate a variety of lean meats, poultry, fish, eggs, dairy products, legumes, nuts, and seeds into your diet.
- Quantity: It is recommended to consume 0.8 grams of protein per kilogram of body weight, taking into account your activity level and individual health requirements.

B. Foods to Add to Your Diet

1. Foods rich in complex carbohydrates:

Complex carbohydrates are digested at a gradual pace, ensuring a consistent and controlled release of glucose into the bloodstream.

- Incorporating whole grains into your diet can be beneficial. Consider adding brown rice, quinoa, whole oats, barley, whole-wheat bread, and pasta to your meals.
- Legumes include beans, lentils, chickpeas, and peas.
- Starchy vegetables include sweet potatoes, squash, and corn.

2. Emphasizing Lean Proteins:

Including lean proteins in your diet can help maintain stable blood sugar levels and provide a longer-lasting feeling of fullness.

- Animal Sources: Choose skinless poultry, lean cuts of beef and pork, fish, and seafood for a healthier option.
- Plant-Based Options: Tofu, tempeh, edamame, beans, and lentils.

3. Incorporating healthy fats into your diet is essential for overall well-being.

Including healthy fats in your diet can provide you with sustained energy and support in keeping your blood sugar levels stable.

- Sources: Include avocado, olive oil, nuts, seeds, and fatty fish such as salmon and mackerel. - Omega-3 Fatty

Acids: These fats can be found in flaxseeds, chia seeds, walnuts, and fatty fish, and they offer extra anti-inflammatory benefits.

4. Incorporating a variety of fruits and vegetables into your diet is essential.

Including fruits and vegetables in your diet is crucial for maintaining good health and managing your blood sugar levels.

- Incorporate a variety of non-starchy vegetables into your diet such as broccoli, spinach, kale, bell peppers, and cauliflower.
- Fruits: Enjoy a variety of delicious and nutritious fruits such as apples, berries, citrus fruits, pears, and kiwi. Emphasize the consumption of whole fruits over fruit juices to optimize your fiber intake.

Foods to Avoid

1. Avoiding Refined Sugars:

Consuming refined sugars can lead to sudden increases and subsequent decreases in blood sugar levels.

- Sources: Sugary beverages, candies, baked goods, and numerous processed foods.

- Other options: Consider incorporating natural sweeteners such as stevia or small amounts of honey into your diet, while remaining mindful of your overall intake.

2. Foods with a High Glycemic Index:

High-GI foods can lead to rapid digestion and result in sudden increases in blood sugar levels.

- Examples: Avoiding foods such as white bread, white rice, pastries, and sugary cereals can be beneficial for your health.
- Consider other options: Opt for whole grain or low-GI alternatives.

3. Be cautious with your caffeine intake:

Excessive consumption of caffeine can contribute to higher blood sugar fluctuations and heightened stress levels, potentially impacting blood sugar management.

- Sources: Coffee, energy drinks, and certain sodas.
- Moderation: It's best to enjoy coffee in moderate amounts, such as 1-2 cups per day. It's also a good idea to avoid adding sugary ingredients to your coffee.

4. Alcohol in Excess:

Consuming too much alcohol can disrupt the regulation of blood sugar levels and potentially cause hypoglycemia, particularly when consumed without eating.

- Recommendation: If you decide to consume alcohol, it is advisable to do so in moderation. According to the guidelines set by the American Diabetes Association, women are advised to limit their alcohol consumption to one drink per day, while men are recommended to have no more than two drinks per day.
- Making Intelligent Decisions: Consider choosing beverages with lower carbohydrate content, such as dry wine or spirits mixed with sugar-free mixers. It is advisable to always consume alcohol with food.

A Practical Diet Plan for Managing Low Blood Sugar Levels

First day:

- Breakfast: Enjoy a delicious bowl of oatmeal with a delightful addition of fresh berries and a touch of chia seeds.
- Snack: Enjoy some delicious apple slices paired with creamy almond butter.

- Lunch: Enjoy a refreshing quinoa salad filled with mixed greens, cherry tomatoes, cucumbers, grilled chicken, and a zesty lemon vinaigrette.
- Snack: Enjoy a nutritious combination of Greek yogurt and a handful of nuts.
- Dinner: Enjoy a delicious meal of baked salmon accompanied by roasted sweet potatoes and steamed broccoli.

Day 2:

- Breakfast: Enjoy a delicious and nutritious meal of whole-grain toast topped with creamy avocado and a perfectly poached egg.
- Snack: Enjoy some nutritious carrot sticks paired with delicious hummus.
- Lunch: Enjoy a nutritious lentil soup accompanied by a side of wholesome whole-grain crackers.
- Snack: Enjoy a refreshing pear paired with a nutritious handful of walnuts.
- Dinner: Enjoy a delicious stir-fried tofu dish accompanied by a colorful medley of mixed vegetables, including bell peppers, broccoli, and snap peas. Served over a bed of nutritious brown rice.

Day 3:

- Breakfast: Start your day with a nutritious smoothie packed with fresh

spinach, ripe banana, protein powder,
and creamy almond milk.
- Snack: Enjoy a nutritious handful of
mixed nuts.
- Lunch: Enjoy a delicious whole-wheat
pita filled with turkey, crisp lettuce, juicy
tomato, and creamy avocado.
- Snack: Enjoy some delicious sliced bell
peppers with a side of creamy guacamole.
- Dinner: Enjoy a delicious meal of grilled
chicken breast paired with quinoa and a
side of roasted Brussels sprouts.

Day 4:

Day 4:

- Breakfast: Enjoy a delicious Greek
yogurt parfait topped with a medley of
fresh berries, crunchy granola, and a
touch of natural sweetness from a drizzle
of honey.
- Snack: Enjoy a delightful combination
of a small handful of almonds and a
piece of rich dark chocolate.
- Lunch: Enjoy a delicious chickpea and
vegetable curry accompanied by
nutritious brown rice.
- Snack: Enjoy a delightful combination
of cottage cheese with juicy pineapple
chunks.
- Dinner: Enjoy a delicious meal of baked
cod accompanied by steamed asparagus

and a refreshing mixed green salad
dressed with olive oil and vinegar.

Day 5:

- For breakfast, enjoy a delicious
combination of scrambled eggs with
nutritious spinach and a side of whole-
grain toast.
- Snack: Enjoy a refreshing combination
of sliced cucumber and cherry tomatoes
paired with tzatziki sauce.
- Lunch: Enjoy a delicious whole-grain
wrap filled with grilled chicken, creamy
avocado, fresh spinach, and a light
dressing.
- Snack: Enjoy some refreshing orange
slices paired with a small handful of
nutritious cashews.
- Dinner: Enjoy a delicious and nutritious
meal of lean beef stir-fry with a colorful
medley of mixed vegetables (bell
peppers, onions, zucchini) served over a
bed of wholesome quinoa.

Day 6:

- Breakfast: Enjoy a delicious smoothie
bowl made with a blend of frozen berries,
banana, and spinach. Top it off with
some crunchy granola and coconut flakes
for added texture and flavor.
- Snack: Enjoy a nutritious combination
of pistachios and an apple.

- Lunch: Enjoy a delicious turkey and avocado salad packed with mixed greens, cherry tomatoes, cucumbers, and a flavorful balsamic vinaigrette.
- Snack: Enjoy a delicious and nutritious combination of whole-grain bread with peanut butter.
- Dinner: Enjoy a delicious meal of grilled shrimp skewers accompanied by a serving of flavorful wild rice and nutritious steamed green beans.

Seventh day:

- Breakfast: Enjoy a nutritious start to your day with a bowl of whole-grain cereal, paired with almond milk and a generous serving of fresh berries. This delicious combination will provide you with the energy you need to kickstart your morning.
- Snack: Enjoy a nutritious combination of a hard-boiled egg and a small handful of mixed nuts.
- Lunch: Enjoy a delicious black bean and quinoa bowl topped with corn, avocado, salsa, and a refreshing squeeze of lime.
- Snack: Enjoy a refreshing fruit salad filled with a delightful assortment of seasonal fruits.
- Dinner: Enjoy a delicious meal of baked chicken thighs accompanied by roasted sweet potatoes and a side of sautéed kale.

Helpful Suggestions for a Diet that Supports Stable Blood Sugar Levels

1. Meal Planning and Preparation: - It's important to plan your meals and snacks in advance so that you always have a variety of balanced options at your fingertips.
    - Cooking meals in larger quantities can help you save time and resist the urge to snack on unhealthy foods.

2. Understanding Food Labels:
    - It is important to carefully examine food labels to identify any additional sugars and opt for products that have minimal or no added sugars.
    - It's important to be mindful of portion sizes and the amount of carbohydrates in each serving.

3. Staying Hydrated: - It is important to make sure you drink an adequate amount of water throughout the day. Thirst and hunger can sometimes be confused.
    As an expert in diabetes, I can provide valuable insights and guidance on managing this condition. With my knowledge and experience, I can help you understand the best strategies for controlling your blood sugar levels and maintaining a healthy lifestyle. Feel free

to ask me any questions It is advisable
to reduce the consumption of sugary
drinks and opt for healthier alternatives
such as water, herbal teas, or other low-
calorie beverages.

4. Healthy Snacking: - Make sure to have
a variety of nutritious snacks available,
like nuts, seeds, fresh fruit, and whole-
grain crackers.
   - It's best to steer clear of processed
snacks that contain excessive amounts of
refined sugars and unhealthy fats.

5. Dining Out: - Opt for restaurants that
provide nutritious choices and seek out
meals that incorporate whole grains, lean
proteins, and ample vegetables.
   - Feel free to request any modifications
you'd like, such as having the dressing
on the side or swapping out fries for a
salad.

A well-balanced diet that promotes stable
blood sugar levels is key for managing
hypoglycemia. This involves eating
regular meals that include high-fiber and
low-GI foods, as well as ensuring
adequate protein intake. By emphasizing
the importance of a balanced diet that
includes complex carbohydrates, lean
proteins, healthy fats, and a wide range
of fruits and vegetables, people can
effectively regulate their blood sugar

levels and avoid episodes of low blood sugar. It is beneficial to steer clear of refined sugars, high-GI foods, excessive caffeine, and alcohol in order to reduce blood sugar fluctuations and promote overall well-being.

By incorporating these dietary principles into your routine, along with consistent monitoring and making necessary lifestyle adjustments, you can take a comprehensive approach to effectively managing hypoglycemia. Through careful meal planning, diligent reading of food labels, staying properly hydrated, and making wise decisions when dining out, individuals can effectively maintain a well-rounded diet that aligns with their goals of managing blood sugar levels.

CHAPTER 6

7 Days Hypoglycemia Diet Plan

Creating a diet plan to manage low blood sugar requires thoughtful attention to balancing nutrients and timing meals to keep blood sugar levels stable throughout the day. Here's a detailed 7-day plan that offers a wide range of nutritious meals and snacks to help you maintain optimal blood sugar control:

Day 1

1. Start your day with a nutritious breakfast of Greek yogurt topped with fresh berries and a sprinkle of oats.
As an experienced professional in the field of diabetes, I can provide valuable insights and guidance on managing this condition. With my expertise, I can help you navigate the challenges associated with diabetes and develop a personalized plan for your health. Let's work together

to improve Greek yogurt is a great
source of protein and probiotics, while
berries provide a healthy dose of
antioxidants and fiber. Oats provide a
source of complex carbohydrates that
can help sustain energy levels.

2. Snack: Enjoy some apple slices paired
with almond butter
- Apples are a great source of natural
sugars and fiber, while almond butter
provides protein and healthy fats to help
you feel satisfied.

3. Lunch: Enjoy a delicious and nutritious
quinoa salad packed with chickpeas and
a variety of fresh vegetables. Quinoa is a
nutritious grain that is rich in protein. It
can be paired with chickpeas to enhance
the protein and fiber content of your
meal. Adding mixed vegetables to your
diet can provide you with a variety of
essential vitamins and minerals.

4. Snack: Enjoy some carrot sticks with a
delicious hummus dip. Carrots are
packed with beta-carotene and fiber,
making them a nutritious choice. On the
other hand, hummus provides a good
source of protein and healthy fats.

5. Dinner: Healthy Meal Option - Enjoy a
delicious grilled chicken dish
accompanied by steamed broccoli and

brown rice. This meal provides lean protein, fiber, vitamins, and complex carbs.

Day 2

1. Start your day with a nutritious breakfast: Scrambled eggs with spinach and whole grain toast. Adding eggs to your diet can provide you with a good source of protein and healthy fats, while incorporating spinach into your meals can help you get essential vitamins and minerals. Whole grain toast is a great source of complex carbohydrates.

2. Snack: Cottage Cheese with Pineapple Chunks - Cottage cheese is a great source of protein and calcium, while pineapple adds a touch of natural sweetness and a boost of vitamin C.

3. Lunch: Delicious Turkey and Avocado Wrap - Turkey is a fantastic source of lean protein, especially when paired with creamy avocado for a dose of healthy fats and wrapped in a whole grain wrap for a satisfying serving of complex carbs.

4. Snack: Mixed Nuts - Nuts provide a good source of protein, healthy fats, and fiber to help you feel satisfied and maintain stable blood sugar levels.

5. Dinner: Enjoy a delicious and nutritious meal of baked salmon paired with sweet potato and asparagus.- Salmon is a great source of omega-3 fatty acids and protein, which makes it a healthy choice. You can pair it with sweet potato to get complex carbs and asparagus to add fiber and vitamins to your meal.

Day 3

1. Start your day with a nutritious breakfast: Enjoy a delicious bowl of oatmeal topped with fresh banana slices and a sprinkle of chia seeds. Including oatmeal, banana, and chia seeds in your diet can provide a balanced mix of complex carbs, fiber, natural sugars, and omega-3 fatty acids.

2. Snack: Greek Yogurt with Honey - Greek yogurt offers a good source of protein and probiotics, complemented by the natural sweetness of honey.

3. Enjoy a delicious lunch of lentil soup accompanied by a refreshing side salad. - Lentils provide a good source of protein and fiber, which can be complemented by a side salad to ensure a well-rounded meal with essential vitamins and minerals.

4. Snack: Nutritious Celery Sticks with a Delicious Peanut Butter Twist - Celery is a great source of fiber and hydration, while peanut butter adds a boost of protein and nourishing fats.

5. Dinner: Delicious Stir-Fried Tofu with Vegetables and Quinoa - Tofu is a great source of plant-based protein, which is perfectly complemented by the fiber-rich vegetables and the complex carbs from quinoa.

Day 4

1. Start your day with a nutritious smoothie that includes spinach, berries, and protein powder.- Spinach is a great source of vitamins and minerals, while berries offer a healthy dose of antioxidants. Additionally, protein powder can help with muscle repair and keeping you feeling satisfied.

2. Snack: A small portion of trail mix - Trail mix provides a combination of nuts, seeds, and dried fruits that are rich in protein, beneficial fats, and naturally occurring sugars.

3. Lunch: Grilled Chicken Caesar Salad - Enjoy a delicious and nutritious grilled chicken Caesar salad, featuring protein-packed grilled chicken, fiber-rich romaine

lettuce, and a light Caesar dressing for added flavor.

4. Snack: Sliced Bell Peppers with Guacamole - Bell peppers are a great source of vitamin C and fiber, while guacamole is packed with healthy fats and fiber.

5. Dinner: Spaghetti Squash with Turkey Meatballs - Enjoy a delicious and healthy dinner with this spaghetti squash dish. The low-carb squash pairs perfectly with flavorful turkey meatballs and marinara sauce.

Day 5

1. Start Your Day with a Nutritious Breakfast: Whole Grain Waffles with Fresh Fruit - Enjoy a delicious and wholesome breakfast option by choosing whole grain waffles. These waffles are packed with complex carbohydrates and fiber, providing you with sustained energy throughout the morning. Top them off with fresh fruit for a burst of natural sugars and essential vitamins to kickstart your day.

2. Snack: Yogurt with Flaxseeds - Yogurt provides protein and probiotics, while flaxseeds offer omega-3 fatty acids and fiber.

3. Lunch: Nutritious Bean and Vegetable Burrito - This delicious burrito is packed with protein and fiber from beans, as well as essential vitamins and minerals from a variety of vegetables. It is all wrapped up in a wholesome whole grain tortilla, providing you with complex carbohydrates to keep you energized.

4. Snack: Enjoy some grapes and cheese cubes. Grapes are a great source of natural sugars and antioxidants, while cheese is rich in protein and calcium.

5. Dinner: Enjoy a delicious and nutritious meal of baked cod served with brown rice and green beans.
As an experienced professional in the field of diabetes, I can provide valuable insights and guidance on managing this condition. With my expertise, I can help you navigate the challenges and make informed decisions to improve your health. Let's work together to develop a personalized plan Enjoy a nutritious meal with cod, a great source of lean protein and omega-3 fatty acids. Pair it with brown rice for a boost of complex carbs and green beans for added fiber and vitamins.

Day 6
1. Start your day with a delicious Chia

Pudding topped with fresh mango. It's a nutritious and satisfying breakfast option.

- Chia pudding is a nutritious choice, providing omega-3 fatty acids and fiber. It's even better when topped with mango, which adds a touch of natural sweetness and a dose of vitamins.

2. Snack: Hard-boiled Egg with a Slice of Avocado
Sorry, I cannot provide a response without any text to work with. Please provide some information or a question so that I can assist you. Eggs are a great source of protein and healthy fats, and avocado adds even more healthy fats and fiber to your diet.

3. Lunch: Enjoy a delicious and nutritious Chicken and Vegetable Stir-Fry.
- Chicken is a great source of protein, which is complemented by a mix of vegetables to add fiber and a stir-fry sauce to enhance the flavor.
4. Snack Idea: Enjoying a nutritious combination of an apple and a handful of walnuts. Apples are a great source of natural sugars and fiber, while walnuts are packed with protein, healthy fats, and omega-3 fatty acids.

5. Dinner: Hearty Beef and Vegetable Stew - This delicious stew combines

tender beef with a variety of vegetables, creating a nutritious and satisfying meal that is perfect for a cozy evening.

 Good day 7

1. Breakfast: Nutritious Smoothie Bowl with Almond Butter and Granola - Start your day with a delicious smoothie bowl packed with a variety of fruits, vegetables, and protein. Enhance the flavor with a dollop of almond butter for a dose of healthy fats and add some granola for an extra crunch.

2. Snack: Edamame - Edamame is a great choice for a nutritious snack, as it offers plant-based protein and fiber.

3. Lunch: Enjoy a delicious and nutritious Quinoa and Black Bean Salad. Quinoa is a great source of protein and complex carbs, which are complemented by the addition of black beans for extra protein and fiber. The dish is then mixed with a variety of vegetables and a light dressing.

4. Snack: Enjoy a refreshing combination of juicy orange slices and creamy cottage cheese.
Can you provide me with some information about diabetes? Oranges are a great source of natural sugars and

vitamin C, while cottage cheese is packed with protein and calcium.

5. Dinner: Enjoy a delicious meal of shrimp and vegetable skewers served with a side of couscous.
- Shrimp is a great source of lean protein and omega-3 fatty acids, which can be complemented by a variety of vegetables to increase fiber intake. Pairing it with couscous adds complex carbohydrates to the meal.

This 7-day diet plan provides a range of nutritious meals and snacks to help maintain stable blood sugar levels throughout the day. By emphasizing the importance of a diet rich in whole, unprocessed foods that offer a variety of nutrients, individuals can effectively control their blood sugar levels while still enjoying tasty and fulfilling meals. In addition, it is crucial to maintain proper hydration, engage in regular physical activity, and diligently monitor blood sugar levels as advised by a healthcare professional. These factors play a vital role in effectively managing blood sugar levels.

THE END